Keto Mexican Cookbook

77 Recipes for Tasty and Spicy High Protein Low Carbs Mexican Food at Home.

**BELINDA
TURNER**

Table of Contents

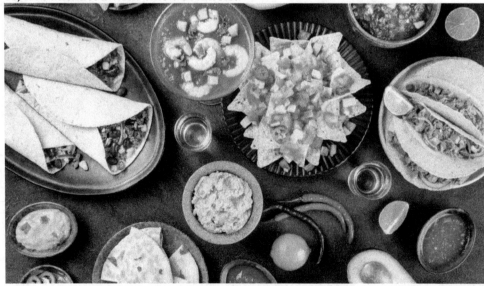

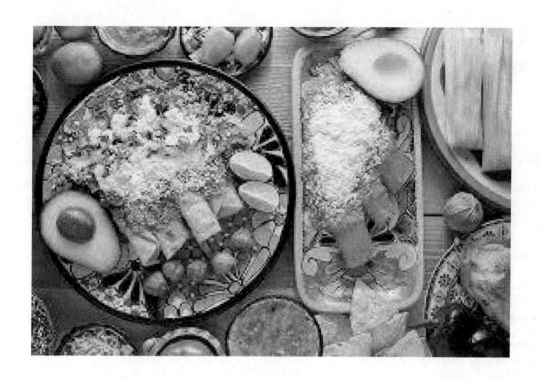

Table of contents

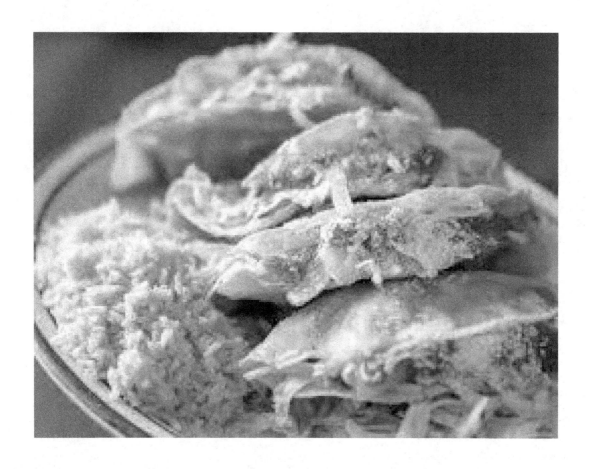

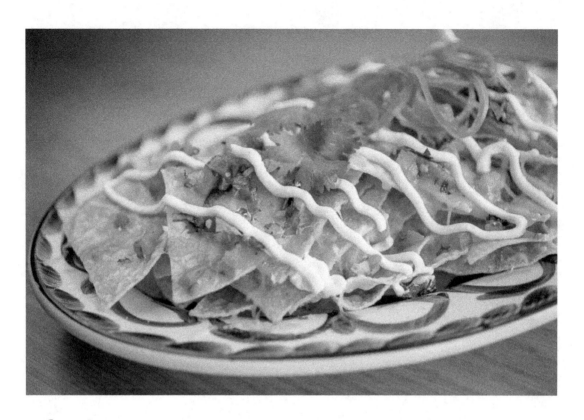

Introduction

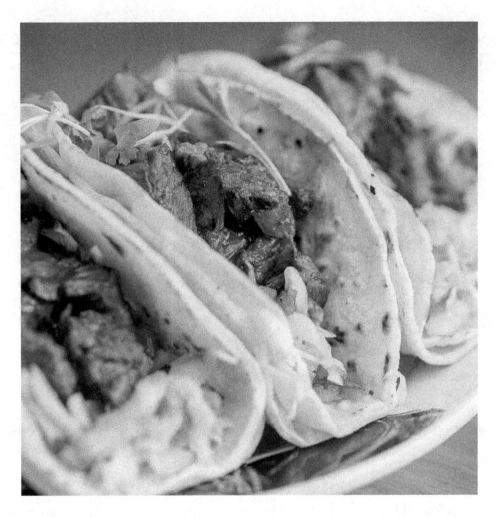

Mexican food comprises of the cooking styles and customs of the territory of Mexico. Its underlying foundations lie in a blend of Mesoamerican and Spanish food. A large number of its fixings and techniques have their foundations in the primary farming networks. Contrasted with numerous different sorts of cooking in Mexico, the food that is found in Mexico City is similarly as amazing as the individuals who have moved there.

Mexican food is well known all around the globe. From tacos to enchiladas and nachos, Mexican impact in cooking can be found anywhere. The locals of Mexico value utilizing normal, organic ingredients. Today, the greater part of what we see as credible Mexican food is really a mix of Mexican food that has been Americanized, generally beginning around the southern fringe of Texas and Mexico.

In this book you will learn Keto Mexican recipes for the people who are either on a Keto diet or want to start it or have any medical condition that requires them to move towards Keto diet. You will find 77 recipes that consist of Keto breakfast, lunch, dinner, snacks, and most importantly vegetarian recipes that you can easily follow to have your Mexican food prepared right in your kitchen. So, you do not have to wait any further, start cooking now!

Chapter 1: Welcome to the World of Keto Mexican Breakfast Recipes

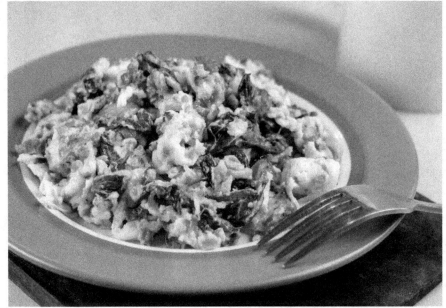

Breakfasts are a start to you day, if you eat healthy and fresh in the beginning of your day it is guaranteed that you would feel the same throughout the course of the day. Keto Mexican breakfasts are very easy to make if you follow the easy recipes that have been mentioned below:

1.1 Keto Mexican Scramble Eggs

Cooking Time: 10 minutes

Serving: 3

Ingredients:

- Jalapenos, one
- Tomato, one
- Eggs, six
- Pepper jack cheese, one cup
- Scallions, half cup
- Salt and pepper
- Butter, one ounce

Instructions:

1. Add the scallions, tomatoes and jalapenos in the butter and let it cook for five minutes.
2. Add the salt and pepper into it.
3. Add the eggs into the mixture.
4. Add pepper jack cheese.

5. Scramble the egg, mix it thoroughly.
6. When your cheese melts, switch off the stove.
7. Your dish is ready to be served.

1.2 Keto Mexican Breakfast Casserole

Cooking Time: 30 minutes
Serving: 6

Ingredients:

- Ground chorizo sauces, one pound
- Minced onion, one
- Eggs, twelve
- Mixed cheese, two cups
- Queso fresco, as required
- Heavy cream, half cup
- Roasted poblano pepper, half cup
- Garlic salt, one tsp.
- Diced tomatoes, two
- Cayenne pepper, half tsp.
- Cilantro, two tbsp.
- Salt and pepper
- Avocado, one
- Vegetable oil, two tbsp.

Instructions:

1. Add onions in the vegetable oil.
2. Sauté the onions until they are soft, add the tomatoes and cook it properly.
3. Add the ground chorizo sausage into the mixture.
4. Add spices, the roasted poblano pepper, and garlic salt into the mixture.
5. Cook for ten minutes straight.
6. Now remove the pan from stove.
7. Add the egg mixture into the pan and mix it well.
8. Now add the shredded mozzarella cheese on top.
9. Bake it for fifteen to twenty minutes.
10. Add cilantro on top before serving.
11. You can serve it with queso fresco and avocado slices.
12. Your dish is ready to be served.

1.3 Baked Eggs in Avocado

Cooking Time: 15 minutes
Serving: 6

Ingredients:

- Chopped chives, two tbsp.
- Eggs, six

- Salt and pepper
- Avocado, three
- Vegetable oil, two tbsp.

Instructions:
1. Cut the avocados in half.
2. Remove the seed and crack the egg and add it in the seed hole.
3. Add the chopped chives on the avocados.
4. Add salt and pepper and bake for ten minutes.
5. Your dish is ready to be served.

1.4 Migas Breakfast Taco
Cooking Time: 20 minutes
Serving: 4
Ingredients:
- Avocado, one
- Salt, half tsp.
- Black pepper, half tsp.
- Eggs, six
- Tortilla chips, one cup
- Salsa, one cup
- Pepper jack cheese, one cup
- Onion, half cup
- Tortillas, six
- Poblano pepper, one
- Cilantro leaves, a quarter cup

Instructions:
1. Add vegetable oil in a pan.
2. Add the onions, eggs, salt, pepper, poblano pepper, and cilantro.
3. Add the avocados and cook for ten minutes.
4. Add the cheese and lightly fry the tortillas.
5. Arrange all the things in the tortillas and add the crushed tortilla chips on top.
6. Your dish is ready to be served.

1.5 Mexican Keto Pancakes
Cooking Time: 5 minutes
Serving: 2
Ingredients:
- Butter two tbsp.
- Ground husk powder, one tbsp.
- Eggs, four
- Cottage cheese, half cup
- Fresh fruits, as required

Instructions:

1. Mix all the ingredients except the fresh fruits in a bowl.
2. Next, add a little butter on a pan and add the batter on top.
3. Cook the pan cakes until they reach golden brown color.
4. Place the fresh fruits on top.
5. Your dish is ready to be served.

1.6 Mexican Keto Breakfast Bowl

Cooking Time: 15 minutes

Serving: 2

Ingredients:

- Chorizo sausage, half pound
- Eggs, four
- Avocado, as required
- Milk, two tbsp.
- Butter, one tbsp.
- Salsa, as required
- Sour cream, as required

Instructions:

1. Cook the chorizo over a medium heat in a large pan.
2. Place cooked chorizo on a paper towel and pour out some of the grease leaving some to cook the eggs in.
3. Break two eggs into a medium heat skillet with chorizo grease and scramble.
4. Add milk if desired to make it fluffier.
5. Once cooked place eggs at the bottom of a bowl.
6. Top the eggs with the cooked chorizo and other toppings that you desire to add.
7. Your dish is ready to be served.

1.7 Mexican Keto Breakfast Hash

Cooking Time: 25 minutes

Serving: 2

Ingredients:

- Chorizo sausage, half pound
- Eggs, two
- Avocado, as required
- Tomatoes, one
- Onion, one
- Zucchini, one
- Salt and pepper, as desired
- Cilantro, as desired
- Butter, one tbsp.
- Avocado slices, as required

Instructions:

1. Add butter to the pan and then add in the onions.
2. Cook the onions for two minutes approximately and then add the peppers into it.
3. Next, add the zucchini and tomatoes.
4. Cook the mixture for about two minutes and then add the chorizo sausage.
5. After adding the chorizo, let it cook for five minutes.
6. Create two holes with the help of a spoon in the mixture.
7. Add the eggs into the holes.
8. Add salt and pepper as desired.
9. Broil the mixture for five minutes until the egg looks cooked properly.
10. Remove from the broiler and add cilantro and avocado slices on top.
11. Your dish is ready to be served.

1.8 Keto Breakfast Taco

Cooking Time: 10 minutes

Serving: 6

Ingredients:

- Cheddar cheese half cup
- Mozzarella cheese, half cup
- Avocado, one
- Salt and pepper, as desired
- Eggs, six
- Taco shells, six
- Butter, two tbsp.
- Bacon, six strips

Instructions:

1. Add the butter on the pan and cook the bacon sheets.
2. Lightly heat the taco shells.
3. Cook the eggs, add the salt and pepper on it and scramble it.
4. Add the egg mixture on the taco shells; add the bacon strips on each.
5. Add the cheese and bake the taco shells for five minutes.
6. Add the avocado slices on top when the tacos are done.
7. Your dish is ready to be served

1.9 Keto Chorizo Eggs

Cooking Time: 10 minutes

Serving: 6

Ingredients:

- Avocado oil, one tbsp.
- Avocado, one
- Salt and pepper, as desired

- Eggs, six
- Avocado, one
- Cilantro, as desired
- Ground chorizo, half pound

Instructions:
1. Add the onions in a pan with the avocado oil.
2. Cook the ground chorizo and mix it until it is properly cooked.
3. Add the salt and pepper on top.
4. Pour in the eggs into the mixture and cook it properly.
5. Add the cilantro and avocado on top of the mixture.
6. Your dish is ready to be served.

1.10 Keto Chilaquiles

Cooking Time: 20 minutes

Serving: 4

Ingredients:
- Coconut oil, two tbsp.
- Shredded cheese, half cup
- Sliced scallions, one
- Sour cream, two tbsp.
- Pork rinds, one pound
- Red salsa, one cup
- Eggs, two
- Salt and pepper, to taste
- Hot sauce, as required
- Cilantro, as required
- Tortillas, as required

Instructions:
1. Add the coconut oil in a pan.
2. Add the pork rinds and cook for ten minutes straight.
3. Add the eggs and scramble until set.
4. Add salt and pepper and then transfer the egg and pork rinds mixture into a baking dish.
5. Add the shredded cheese and bake for five minutes.
6. Add cilantro on top and serve with hot sauce, red salsa, and tortillas.

1.11 Keto Huevos Rancheros

Cooking Time: 15 minutes

Serving: 4

Ingredients:
- Mexican cheese, two cups
- Eggs, four

- Cilantro, as required
- Coconut oil, one tbsp.
- Salt and pepper, as required
- Lime, as required
- Red salsa, one cup

Instructions:
1. Add the coconut oil in a pan.
2. Add in the cheese, blend and let it melt.
3. Add the egg on top and sprinkle salt and pepper on top.
4. Cover with a lid for five minutes.
5. Now, add cilantro on top.
6. Add the lime wedges and salsa on the side.
7. Your dish is ready to be served.

1.12 Keto Breakfast Burrito

Cooking Time: 15 minutes

Serving: 4

Ingredients:
- Refried beans, one cup
- Cooked ground beef, one pound
- Scrambled eggs, eight
- Salt and pepper, to taste
- Hot sauce, as required
- Minced garlic, three
- Mixed cheese, one cup
- Avocado, one
- Jalapeno, one
- Tortillas, four
- Tomatoes, one

Instructions:
1. In the center of each tortilla, spread the refried beans; add the ground beef, the scrambled eggs, add the taco seasoning, some cheese, and tomato pieces, jalapeno, and avocado.
2. Fold in the two sides and roll up tightly.
3. Lightly fry the burrito.
4. Serve with hot sauce.

Chapter 2: Keto Mexican Lunch Recipes

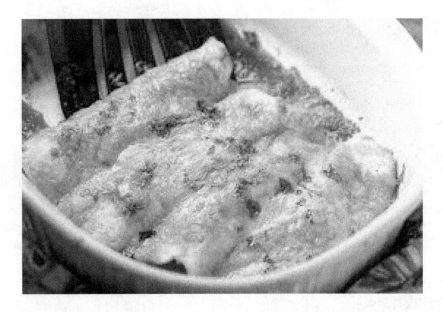

Mexican lunch recipes are very easy to make and especially those recipes that are included into the Keto diet. Following are some amazing Keto lunch recipes:

2.1 Keto Chicken Enchilada

Cooking Time: 18 minutes

Serving: 6

Ingredients:

- Ground chicken meat, one pound
- Salt and pepper, to taste
- Enchilada sauce, as required
- Onion, one
- Minced garlic, three
- Mixed cheese, one cup
- Avocado, one
- Jalapeno, one
- Tortillas, six
- Tomatoes, one
- Vegetable oil, two tbsp.
- Cilantro, as required

Instructions:

1. Add chopped onions in a pan with the vegetable oil.
2. Once the onions are soft, add the garlic into it.
3. Then, add the chicken mince into it.
4. Cook for a few minutes and then add tomatoes and let it simmer for five minutes.
5. Add salt and pepper, mix and set aside.

6. Take the tortilla sheets and add the chicken mixture in the center and roll it.
7. Place the rolled tortillas in a baking dish and pour the enchilada sauce over it.
8. Next add the shredded cheese on top.
9. Bake for five minutes until the cheese is melted.
10. Add the cilantro on top and your dish is ready to be served.

2.2 Keto Chicken Chimichangas

Cooking Time: 10 minutes

Serving: 2

Ingredients:

- Cooked taco ground beef, one cup
- Mixed cheese, one cup
- Salsa, half cup
- Avocado, one
- Jalapeno, one
- Tortillas, six
- Cilantro, as required

Instructions:

1. Add the beef in the tortillas and roll it.
2. Place the tortillas on a baking dish and cover with cheese.
3. Bake for five minutes and then top with cilantro leaves.
4. Add the jalapenos, avocados, and salsa on top.
5. Your dish is ready to be served.

2.3 Keto Mexican Skillet

Cooking Time: 15 minutes

Serving: 6

Ingredients:

- Ground beef meat, one pound
- Diced bell pepper, half
- Salt and pepper, to taste
- Green chilies, half cup
- Taco seasoning, three tbsp.
- Diced onion, one
- Cauliflower rice, one cup
- Sour cream, as required
- Jalapeno, one
- Tortillas, six
- Avocado one
- Avocado oil, two tbsp.
- Cilantro, as required

Instructions:

1. Heat the avocado oil in a skillet.
2. Add in the beef and cook.
3. Add in the onion, bell pepper, and taco seasoning and cook a few minutes or until the onion and pepper start to soften.
4. Stir in the green chilies and tomatoes along with the cauliflower rice.
5. Top with all the toppings.
6. Your dish is ready to be served.

2.4 Keto Meatball Tacos

Cooking Time: 20 minutes
Serving: 4
Ingredients:
- Chopped red onion, half
- Chicken mince, one pound
- Olive oil, five tbsp.
- Taco shells, eight
- Barbeque sauce, two tbsp.
- Chopped avocado, one
- Chopped cilantro, a bunch
- Salt and pepper to taste
- Red paprika powder, two tsp.

Instructions:
1. Add the mince in a bowl with the salt, red paprika, and pepper and mix.
2. Make balls and cook it for ten minutes until done.
3. Now arrange your tacos, add meatballs, barbeque sauce, avocado, onion and cilantro on top.
4. Your dish is ready to be served.

2.5 Keto Mexican Cheesy Chicken Skillet

Cooking Time: 18 minutes
Serving: 6
Ingredients:
- Ground beef meat, one pound
- Diced bell pepper, half
- Salt and pepper, to taste
- Green chilies, half cup
- Taco seasoning, three tbsp.
- Diced onion, one
- Cauliflower rice, one cup
- Sour cream, as required
- Jalapeno, one
- Tortillas, six

- Avocado one
- Cheese blend, one cup
- Avocado oil, two tbsp.
- Cilantro, as required

Instructions:
1. Heat the avocado oil in a skillet.
2. Add in the beef and cook.
3. Add in the onion, bell pepper, and taco seasoning and cook for a few minutes or until the onion and pepper start to soften.
4. Stir in the green chilies and tomatoes along with the cauliflower rice.
5. Add the cheese blend and bake it for five minutes.
6. Top with all the toppings.
7. Your dish is ready to be served.

2.6 Keto Mexican Ground Beef Casseroles

Cooking Time: 35 minutes

Serving: 9

Ingredients:
- Ground beef meat, one pound
- Salt and pepper, to taste
- Sour cream, as required
- Onion, one
- Minced garlic, three cloves
- Mixed cheese, one cup
- Avocado, one
- Jalapeno, one
- Taco seasoning, one tbsp.
- Tortillas, nine
- Tomatoes, one
- Mix vegetables, half cup
- Vegetable oil, two tbsp.
- Cilantro, as required

Instructions:
1. Add the vegetable oil and cook the onions in a pan.
2. Then add the garlic and ground beef.
3. Cook well and add tomatoes, taco seasoning, salt, and pepper into the mixture.
4. Add the mix vegetables and cook for two minutes.
5. Transfer the mixture into a baking dish and top with cheese blend.
6. Bake it for five minutes.
7. Add the cilantro on top and serve it with tortillas and desired toppings.

2.7 Keto Mexican Cauli Rice

Cooking Time: 10 minutes
Serving: 4
Ingredients:
- Ground cauliflower, one large
- Mix spice, one tbsp.
- Salt and pepper, to taste
- Vegetable oil, two tbsp.
- Cilantro, as required

Instructions:
1. Add the vegetable oil in a pan
2. Add the shredded cauliflower into it.
3. Add mix spice into the mixture and cook for two minutes.
4. Next, add salt and pepper and cook it for five minutes.
5. Garnish it with cilantro leaves.
6. Your dish is ready to be served.

2.8 Keto Cabbage Taco Soup
Cooking Time: 15 minutes
Serving: 2
Ingredients:
- Cabbage, two cups
- Salt and pepper, to taste
- Taco seasoning, one tbsp.
- Onion, one
- Minced garlic, three
- Tomatoes, one
- Vegetable oil, two tbsp.
- Cilantro, as required
- Vegetable stock, two cups

Instructions:
1. Add the vegetable oil in a large pan and add the onions.
2. Cook the onions and add garlic into it.
3. Next add tomatoes and then the spices.
4. Add the cauliflower and cook for five minutes.
5. Add the vegetable stock into the mixture.
6. Let it simmer for ten minutes and then add cilantro on top.
7. Your dish is ready to be served.

2.9 Bacon Wrapped Jalapeno Poppers
Cooking Time: 15 minutes
Serving: 6
Ingredients:

- Shredded cheese, half cup
- Jalapeno peppers, twelve
- Bacon strips, twelve
- Cream cheese, one cup
- Cilantro, as required
- Salt and pepper, to taste

Instructions:
1. Add the shredded cheese and cream cheese in a bowl.
2. Mix properly and add the salt and pepper.
3. Add the mixture into the jalapeno peppers and cover it with bacon strips.
4. Bake the poppers for five minutes.
5. Add cilantro on top and serve with your desired sauce.

2.10 Keto Mexican Cauliflower Skewers

Cooking Time: 10 minutes

Serving: 4

Ingredients:
- Wooden skewers, four
- Cauliflower florets, two cups
- Cotija and parmesan cheese, half cup
- Chipotle powder, two tsp.
- Salt, as required
- Chopped cilantro, half cup
- Mayonnaise, half cup
- Red sauce, two tsp.

Instructions:
1. Add the cauliflower florets in skewers.
2. Combine the mayonnaise and red sauce, and then brush generously onto the cauliflower.
3. Sprinkle on all sides with the chipotle powder and salt.
4. Sprinkle or roll in the crumbled cotija or parmesan cheese.
5. Garnish with chopped cilantro.
6. Add the lime juice on top.
7. Your dish is ready to be served.

2.11 Keto Beef Taquitos

Cooking Time: 15 minutes

Serving: 4

Ingredients:
- Ground beef meat, one pound
- Salt and pepper, to taste
- Onion, one

- Minced garlic, three
- Mixed cheese, two cups
- Tortillas, six
- Tomatoes, one
- Vegetable oil, two tbsp.
- Cilantro, as required

Instructions:
1. Add the vegetable oil in a pan and then add onions into the pan.
2. Add the garlic into it and then the beef.
3. Cook properly.
4. Then, add the tomatoes and spices.
5. Cook the mixture for ten minutes.
6. Next in a nonstick pan add cheese in four different places in circles.
7. When it melts add a spoon of the beef mixture and roll the cheese slices.
8. Cook for two minutes.
9. Add cilantro on top and serve it with your preferred sauce.
10. Your dish is ready to be served.

2.12 Baked Cauliflower Tortillas

Cooking Time: 20 minutes
Serving: 6

Ingredients:
- Ground cauliflower, two cups
- Eggs, two
- Salt and pepper, to taste
- Vegetable oil, four tbsp.
- Cilantro, as required

Instructions:
1. Mix all the above ingredients together in a bowl.
2. Add vegetable oil into the pan.
3. Add cauliflower mixture and cook for ten minutes.
4. Cook until golden brown from both sides.
5. You can serve it with your preferred dip.
6. Your dish is ready to be served.

2.13 Keto Chili Corn Carne

Cooking Time: 30 minutes
Serving: 4

Ingredients:

- Chopped chilies, three
- Chili powder, one tsp.
- Salt and pepper, to taste
- Cooked corns, two cups
- Onion, one
- Minced garlic, three
- Paprika, one tsp.
- Coriander powder, one tsp.
- Cumin powder, one tsp.
- Tomato paste, half cup
- Vegetable oil, two tbsp.
- Tomatoes, one
- Cilantro, as required

Instructions:

1. Place a large saucepan over high heat.
2. Add the oil, onions, garlic and chopped chilis into the pan.
3. Add the chili powder and salt into the pan.
4. Add the cooked corn.
5. Sauté for ten minutes until the beef is well browned.
6. Add the tomato paste, paprika, cumin and coriander and stir well.
7. Cook for five minutes before adding the canned diced tomatoes.
8. Reduce the heat to a low simmer and continue to cook for twenty to thirty minutes.
9. Taste your chili.
10. Add additional salt and pepper if desired.
11. Add cilantro on top.
12. Your dish is ready to be served.

2.14 Keto Steak Fajitas

Cooking Time: 12 minutes

Serving: 4

Ingredients:

- Fajita seasoning, four tbsp.
- Beef steak, two pounds
- Mixed bell peppers, three
- Red onions, one
- Olive oil, as required
- Cilantro, as required

Instructions:

1. Add all the ingredients in a bowl and mix properly.

2. Next, grill all the things and cook for ten to twelve minutes approximately.
3. Add cilantro to garnish your meal.
4. Your meal is ready to be served.

2.15 Keto Pork Chops

Cooking Time: 25 minutes
Serving: 4

Ingredients:

- Pork chops, one pound
- Butter, two tbsp.
- Salt and pepper to taste
- Mexican spices two tbsp.
- Broth, one cup
- Cream, two tbsp.
- Cilantro, as required

Instructions:

1. Add the butter into a pan.
2. Then add the pork chops and salt as well as pepper into it.
3. Add cream into the mixture and then add Mexican spices.
4. Add broth into the mixture.
5. Add cilantro on top.
6. Your dish is ready to be served.

Chapter 3: Keto Mexican Dinner Recipes

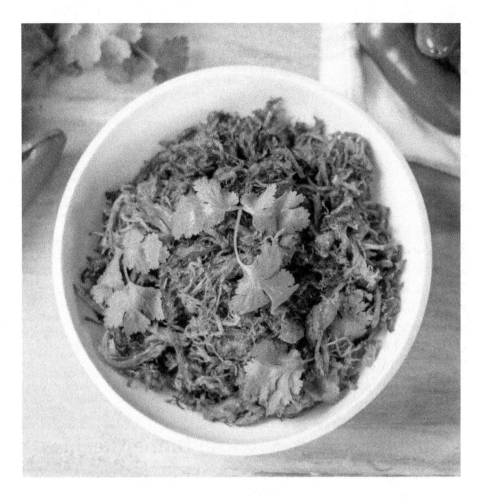

Mexican dinners are very lavish and full of flavors. Following are some amazing Mexican dinner recipes that you can make at home:

3.1 Keto Mexican Pulled Pork

Cooking Time: six hours

Serving: 4

Ingredients:

- Chopped red onion, half
- Pork shoulder, two pounds
- Olive oil, five tbsp.
- Chopped avocado, one
- Chopped cilantro, a bunch
- Salsa, half cup
- Oregano, two tsp.
- Cumin, two tbsp.
- Salt and pepper to taste
- Tortillas, six

Instructions:
1. Add the oregano, salt, cumin, pepper, and pork shoulder.
2. Cook for six hours straight.
3. Shred the pork slices and arrange the tortillas.
4. Add the rest of the ingredients on top.
5. Your dish is ready to be served.

3.2 Keto Prawn Enchiladas

Cooking Time: 18 minutes

Serving: 6

Ingredients:
- Ground prawn meat, one pound
- Salt and pepper, to taste
- Enchilada sauce, as required
- Onion, one
- Minced garlic, three
- Mixed cheese, one cup
- Avocado, one
- Jalapeno, one
- Tortillas, six
- Tomatoes, one
- Vegetable oil, two tbsp.
- Cilantro, as required

Instructions:
1. Add chopped onions in a pan with the vegetable oil.
2. Once the onions are soft, add the garlic into it.
3. Then, add the prawn mince into it.
4. Cook for a few minutes and then add tomatoes and let it simmer for five minutes.
5. Add salt and pepper, mix and set aside.
6. Take the tortilla sheets and add the prawn mixture in the center and roll it.
7. Place the rolled tortillas in a baking dish and pour the enchilada sauce over it.
8. Next add the shredded cheese on top.
9. Bake for five minutes until the cheese is melted.
10. Add the cilantro on top and your dish is ready to be served.

3.3 Keto Chicken Verde Taco Bowls

Cooking Time: 30 minutes

Serving: 6

Ingredients:
- Cauliflower rice, six cups
- Chicken, two pounds

- Salt and pepper, as required
- Taco seasoning, two tbsp.
- Tomatillo sauce, one cup
- Red salsa, as required
- Cilantro, as required
- Vegetable oil, two tbsp.

Instructions:
1. Add the oil and chicken into a pan.
2. Cook the chicken properly.
3. Next add the taco seasoning, salt and pepper into it.
4. In the end add the tomatillo sauce and cook for ten minutes.
5. Then, arrange the cauliflower rice in six different bowls.
6. Add the chicken mixture on top of it.
7. Garnish it with cilantro leaves, and red salsa on top.
8. Your dish is ready to be served.

3.4 Turkey Lettuce Wrap Tacos

Cooking Time: 15 minutes

Serving: 4

Ingredients:
- Turkey meat, one pound
- Butter, two tbsp.
- Salt and pepper to taste
- Mexican spices two tbsp.
- Lettuce wraps, eight
- Cilantro, as required

Instructions:
1. Add the butter and turkey meat in a pan and cook.
2. Add the spices and cook properly.
3. Add cilantro on top.
4. Next, add the mixture into the lettuce wraps and roll it.
5. Your dish is ready to be served with your favorite dip.

3.5 Keto Quesadillas

Cooking Time: 10 minutes

Serving: 4

Ingredients:
- Cooked spinach, two cups
- Butter, two tbsp.
- Salt and pepper to taste
- Mexican spices two tbsp.
- Cheese, one cup

- Tortillas, eight

Instructions:
1. Add the butter in a pan and then add spinach.
2. Add rest of the spices and cook properly.
3. In another pan add the tortillas and add the spinach mixture on top.
4. Then, add the cheese on it.
5. Place another tortilla on top.
6. Cook on both sides.
7. Your dish is ready to be served with your preferred dip.

3.6 Keto Beef and Cheese Chili Bake

Cooking Time: 30 minutes

Serving: 4

Ingredients:
- Chopped chilies, three
- Chili powder, one tsp.
- Salt and pepper, to taste
- Shredded beef, one pound
- Onion, one
- Minced garlic, three
- Paprika, one tsp.
- Coriander powder, one tsp.
- Cumin powder, one tsp.
- Tomato paste, half cup
- Vegetable oil, two tbsp.
- Tomatoes, one
- Cilantro, as required

Instructions:
1. Place a large saucepan over high heat.
2. Add the oil, onions, garlic and chopped chilies into the pan.
3. Add the chili powder and salt into the pan.
4. Add the shredded beef.
5. Sauté for ten minutes until the beef is well browned.
6. Add the tomato paste, paprika, cumin and coriander and stir well.
7. Cook for five minutes before adding the canned diced tomatoes.
8. Reduce the heat to a low simmer and continue to cook for twenty to thirty minutes.
9. Taste your chili.
10. Add additional salt and pepper if desired.
11. Add cheese on top and bake for five minutes.
12. Add cilantro on top.

13. Your dish is ready to be served.

3.7 Keto Green Chili Chicken Enchiladas

Cooking Time: 18 minutes

Serving: 6

Ingredients:

- Ground chicken meat, one pound
- Green chili sauce, two tbsp.
- Salt and pepper, to taste
- Enchilada sauce, as required
- Onion, one
- Minced garlic, three
- Mixed cheese, one cup
- Avocado, one
- Jalapeno, one
- Tortillas, six
- Vegetable oil, two tbsp.
- Cilantro, as required

Instructions:

1. Add chopped onions in a pan with the vegetable oil.
2. Once the onions are soft, add the garlic into it.
3. Then, add the chicken mince into it.
4. Add the green chili sauce into it.
5. Cook for five to ten minutes.
6. Add salt and pepper, mix and set aside.
7. Take the tortilla sheets and add the prawn mixture in the center and roll it.
8. Place the rolled tortillas in a baking dish and pour the enchilada sauce over it.
9. Next add the shredded cheese on top.
10. Bake for five minutes until the cheese is melted.
11. Add the cilantro on top and your dish is ready to be served.

3.8 Keto Tex- Mex Casserole

Cooking Time: 35 minutes

Serving: 9

Ingredients:

- Ground beef meat, one pound
- Salt and pepper, to taste
- Sour cream, as required
- Onion, one
- Minced garlic, three
- Mixed cheese, one cup
- Avocado, one

- Jalapeno, one
- Tex- Mex seasoning, one tbsp.
- Tortillas, nine
- Tomatoes, one
- Mix vegetables, half cup
- Vegetable oil, two tbsp.
- Cilantro, as required

Instructions:
1. Add the vegetable oil and cook the onions in a pan.
2. Then add the garlic and ground beef.
3. Cook well and add tomatoes, Tex- Mex seasoning, salt, and pepper into the mixture.
4. Add the mix vegetables and cook for two minutes.
5. Transfer the mixture into a baking dish and top with cheese blend.
6. Bake it for five minutes.
7. Add the cilantro on top and serve it with tortillas and desired toppings.

3.9 Keto Carne Asada with Chimichurri
Cooking Time: 25 minutes
Serving: 4
Ingredients:
- Pork mince, one pound
- Butter, two tbsp.
- Corn, one cup
- Salt and pepper to taste
- Mexican spices two tbsp.
- Broth, one cup
- Chimichurri sauce, two tbsp.
- Cilantro, as required
- Tortillas, as required

Instructions:
1. Add the butter and pork mince.
2. Cook and add the spices into it.
3. Add the broth and let it cook for fifteen minutes.
4. Then add the chimichurri sauce and corn.
5. Cook for five minutes and then dish out.
6. Garnish it with cilantro.
7. Your dish is ready to be served with tortillas.

3.10 Keto Cheesy Casserole
Cooking Time: 35 minutes
Serving: 9

Ingredients:
- Salt and pepper, to taste
- Sour cream, as required
- Onion, one
- Minced garlic, three
- Mixed cheese, one cup
- Avocado, one
- Jalapeno, one
- Taco seasoning, one tbsp.
- Tortillas, nine
- Tomatoes, one
- Mix vegetables, half cup
- Vegetable oil, two tbsp.
- Cilantro, as required

Instructions:
1. Add the vegetable oil and cook the onions in a pan.
2. Add the minced garlic and cook.
3. Cook well and add tomatoes, taco seasoning, salt, and pepper into the mixture.
4. Add the mix vegetables and cook for two minutes.
5. Transfer the mixture into a baking dish and top with cheese blend.
6. Bake it for five minutes.
7. Add the cilantro on top and serve it with tortillas and desired toppings.

3.11 Keto Mexican Meatloaf

Cooking Time: 25 minutes

Serving: 4

Ingredients:
- Ground beef, one pound
- Butter, two tbsp.
- Cilantro, as required
- Mexican spice mix, two tbsp.
- Tomatoes, two
- Onion, one
- Egg, one
- Salt and pepper, to taste

Instructions:
1. Mix all the ingredients together in a bowl.
2. Add the egg into the mixture.
3. The egg is used for binding the mixture properly.
4. Next place the meat loaf in a baking dish.
5. Cover it all over with butter.

6. Bake for twenty minutes.
7. Cut into slices and serve it with your preferred sauce.

3.12 Keto Mexican Shredded Chicken

Cooking Time: 20 minutes

Serving: 4

Ingredients:

- Shredded chicken, one pound
- Butter, two tbsp.
- Salt and pepper to taste
- Mexican spices two tbsp.
- Broth, one cup
- Cilantro, as required
- Tortillas, as needed
- Tomato paste, half cup

Instructions:

1. In a pan add the butter.
2. Add in the shredded chicken and cook it for a while.
3. Then, add the salt, pepper, and Mexican spice.
4. Next add the tomato paste and mix properly.
5. Add the broth and let it cook for fifteen minutes.
6. Top it with cilantro.
7. Your dish is ready to be served with tortillas.

3.13 Cheesy Beef Taco Skillet

Cooking Time: 15 minutes

Serving: 6

Ingredients:

- Ground beef meat, one pound
- Diced bell pepper, half
- Salt and pepper, to taste
- Green chilies, half cup
- Taco seasoning, three tbsp.
- Diced onion, one
- Cauliflower rice, one cup
- Sour cream, as required
- Jalapeno, one
- Tortillas, six
- Avocado one
- Mixed cheese, one cup
- Avocado oil, two tbsp.
- Cilantro, as required

Instructions:

1. Heat the avocado oil in a skillet.
2. Add in the beef and cook.
3. Add in the onion, bell pepper, and taco seasoning and cook a few minutes or until the onion and pepper starts to soften.
4. Stir in the green chilies and tomatoes along with the cauliflower rice.
5. Add the cheese on top.
6. Bake for five minutes and take it out from the oven.
7. Top with all the toppings.
8. Your dish is ready to be served.

3.14 Keto Chili Rellenos

Cooking Time: 15 minutes

Serving: 4

Ingredients:

- Shredded cheese mix, two cups
- Raw egg, two
- Onion powder, half tsp.
- Poblano peppers, eight
- Olive oil, two tbsp.
- Salt and pepper, as required

Instructions:

1. Roast the poblano peppers for five minutes and then stuff it with cheese mix.
2. Beat the eggs until they get fluffy.
3. Next add the spices into the egg mixture.
4. Coat the peppers in the egg mixture.
5. Fry them in olive oil.
6. Your dish is ready to be served with your preferred dip.

3.15 Keto Tamale Pie

Cooking Time: 25 minutes

Serving: 4

Ingredients:

- Green chilies, one
- Melted butter, two tbsp.
- Cream one tbsp.
- Eggs, two
- Cooked chicken, one pound
- Coconut flour, two tbsp.
- Suga substitute, one tbsp.
- Baking soda, one tsp.
- Salt as required

- Enchilada sauce, three tbsp.
- Taco seasoning, two tsp.
- Cheese, one cup
- Cilantro, as required

Instructions:

1. Mix the melted butter, cream, and eggs in a bowl.
2. Add the green chilies, coconut flour, sugar substitute, salt, and baking soda to the bowl and stir well to combine.
3. Spread the mixture into the prepared dish and bake for fifteen minutes.
4. The cornbread should be just set on top, but still somewhat jiggly in the center.
5. Use a fork to poke holes all over the cornbread.
6. Cover the top of the cornbread with the enchilada sauce.
7. Add the cooked chicken and taco seasoning to a bowl and stir to coat.
8. Arrange chicken over the top of the cornbread and sprinkle with grated cheddar.
9. Return to the oven for ten minutes.
10. Add cilantro on top.
11. Your dish is ready to be served.

Chapter 4: Keto Mexican Snack Recipes

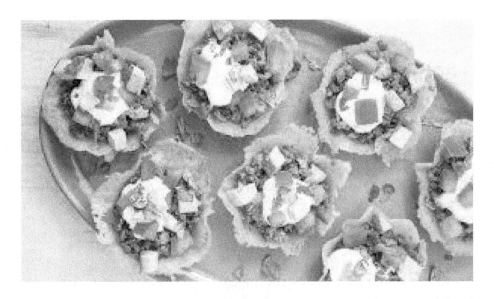

Snacks are loved by everyone; Mexican Keto snacks are extremely delicious and easy to prepare. Following are some Keto Mexican recipes that you can follow:

4.1 Keto Cheese Shell Taco Cups

Cooking Time: 15 minutes

Serving: 4

Ingredients:

- Corn kernels, one cup
- Salt and pepper to taste
- Olive oil, two tbsp.
- Taco spice mix, two tbsp.
- Cilantro, as required
- Green chili sauce, two tbsp.
- Avocado, one
- Shredded cheese, two cups
- Red salsa, as required

Instructions:

1. Add the shredded cheese in the cups of a muffin baking dish and let it bake for five minutes.
2. In a bowl, mix the corn kernels, salt, pepper, taco mix, green chili sauce, and olive oil.
3. Next, add the above made mixture into the shredded cheese cups.
4. Add the cilantro, salsa and avocado slices on top.
5. Your dish is ready to be served.

4.2 Keto Mexican Stuffed Peppers

Cooking Time: 10 minutes

Serving: 4

Ingredients:
- Shredded cheese mix, two cups
- Mix vegetables, one cup
- Onion powder, half tsp.
- Poblano peppers, eight
- Olive oil, two tbsp.
- Salt and pepper, as required

Instructions:
1. Mix the cheese, vegetables and spices together.
2. Stuff it into the poblano peppers and drizzle some olive oil on top.
3. Let it bake for five minutes until the cheese melts.
4. Your dish is ready to be served with your preferred dip or sauce.

4.3 Keto Fat Head Nachos

Cooking Time: 15 minutes
Serving: 4-6

Ingredients:
- Shredded cheese mix, two cups
- Flour, one cup
- Cream cheese, half cup
- Egg, two
- Salt, as required
- Oregano, one tsp.

Instructions:
1. Mix shredded cheese, flour, cream cheese and heat for one minute.
2. Remove from the stove and stir.
3. Add the egg, salt and spices.
4. Place pastry between two parchment rolls into a rectangle.
5. Bake in the oven for twelve minutes until golden brown then flip over and bake until brown.
6. Take out and cut into triangles then bake again for five minutes.
7. Your dish is ready to be served.

4.4 Keto Mexican Pizza

Cooking Time: 15 minutes
Serving: 2

Ingredients:
- Shredded cheese mix, two cups
- Cilantro, as required
- Shredded chicken, one cup
- Jalapenos, two
- Olive oil, two tbsp.

- Salt and pepper, as required

Instructions:
1. Add the cheese on a pan and let it melt.
2. Add the shredded chicken on top.
3. Add jalapeno peppers on top.
4. Add cilantro and olive oil.
5. Your pizza is ready to be served.

4.5 Keto Mexican Chocolate Pudding

Cooking Time: 15 minutes

Serving: 4

Ingredients:
- Cocoa powder, half cup
- Artificial sweetener, half cup
- Vanilla extract, one tsp.
- Cinnamon, half tsp.
- Overripe avocado, one

Instructions:
1. Place all ingredients into a blender and process until smooth.
2. Spoon into two jars and serve immediately or refrigerate.
3. To store, refrigerate the pudding.

4.6 Keto Avocado Ice cream

Cooking Time: 15 minutes

Serving: 4

Ingredients:
- Avocados, four
- Salt, half tsp.
- Unsweetened cocoa powder, two tbsp.
- Coconut milk, one cup
- Vanilla essence, one tsp.
- Erythritol, one tbsp.

Instructions:
1. Open the avocados and remove the flesh into a bowl.
2. Add the avocados into a food processor along with vanilla essence, unsweetened cocoa powder, coconut milk, salt, and erythritol.
3. Blend the mixture for three to five minutes.
4. Always remember the more you blend the fluffier will be the ice cream.
5. Transfer the mixture into a bowl.
6. Freeze at least 1 hour before serving.
7. Serve it with fresh avocados on the side.

4.7 Keto Hot Chocolate Cookies

Cooking Time: 10 minutes
Serving: 8-10
Ingredients:

- Brown sugar, one cup
- Eggs, two
- Baking soda, one tsp.
- Flour, two cups
- Vanilla extract, one tsp.
- Salt, half tsp.
- Unsweetened chocolate chips, one package
- Butter, one cup
- Sugar substitute, half cup
- Unsweetened Cocoa powder, one tbsp.

Instructions:

1. Melt one cup butter.
2. Add half cup sugar substitute and one cup brown sugar.
3. Cream well.
4. Add two teaspoon vanilla extract and two eggs and mix well.
5. Add one teaspoon salt and one teaspoon baking soda and mix together.
6. Mix in the cocoa powder, flour and one package chocolate chips.
7. Roll dough into balls and flatten slightly on cookie sheet.
8. Bake until very light golden brown.
9. To keep cookies moist and soft, do not overbake.

4.8 Keto Creamy Flan

Cooking Time: 50 minutes
Serving: 8-10
Ingredients:

- Erythritol, one tbsp.
- Butter, half cup
- Whipping cream, one cup
- Eggs, four
- Water, two tbsp.

Instructions:

1. In a deep pan, heat up the erythritol for the caramel.
2. Add in the water and butter.
3. Stir occasionally until the sauce becomes golden brown.
4. Pour into the bottom of each ramekin, covering the bottom nicely.
5. In a bowl, mix together the whipping cream, remaining erythritol, and vanilla.
6. In a separate bowl, whisk together the whole eggs.
7. Then add in the yolks, whisking once more.

8. Slowly stir your eggs into the cream mix.
9. Pour the custard into each ramekin on top of the caramel.
10. Place the ramekins into a casserole dish and fill over half way with hot water.
11. Bake for thirty minutes.
12. Take the casserole dish out of the oven but leave the ramekins in the hot water for another ten minutes.
13. When ready to eat, take a knife and slowly run it on the inside of the custard to release it from the ramekin.
14. Your dish is ready to be served.

4.9 Keto Tres Leches Cake

Cooking Time: 25 minutes

Serving: 6

Ingredients:

- Erythritol, one tbsp.
- Eggs, two
- Almond flour, one cup
- Vanilla extract, one tsp.
- Almond milk, one cup
- Baking powder, one tsp.
- Coconut flour, one cup
- Unsweetened condensed milk, half cup
- Heavy cream, two tbsp.
- Whipped cream, as required

Instructions:

1. In a large bowl, beat together the erythritol and butter.
2. Beat in the eggs, one at a time, then the almond milk and vanilla extract.
3. Beat in the almond flour, coconut flour, and baking powder.
4. Transfer the batter to baking pan and smooth the top with a spatula.
5. Bake for twenty minutes, until the top is lightly golden.
6. In a medium bowl, stir together the sweetened condensed milk, almond milk, and heavy cream.
7. Using a fork, poke holes in top of the cake and pour milk mixture over the top.
8. Add whipped cream on top.
9. Your dish is ready to be served.

4.10 Keto Mexican Coffee

Cooking Time: 15 minutes

Serving: 2

Ingredients:

- Cinnamon stick, half
- Cloves, two

- Unsweetened cocoa powder, one tbsp.
- Vanilla extract, half tsp.
- Sugar free brown sugar, two tbsp.
- Erythritol sweetener, one tsp.
- Ground coffee, three tbsp.
- Water, three cups

Instructions:
1. Combine the water, cinnamon, cloves, salt, cocoa powder, and ground coffee in a small saucepan.
2. Bring to a boil and then simmer for five minutes.
3. Remove from the heat and add the vanilla extract, sweetener, and flavored syrup.
4. Stir and then let steep undisturbed for five minutes.
5. Carefully ladle or pour off the coffee into two mugs, leaving the grounds undisturbed at the bottom of the pan.
6. Your dish is ready to be served.

4.11 Keto Paloma Cocktail

Cooking Time: 15 minutes
Serving: 2

Ingredients:
- Artificial sweetener, one tbsp.
- Grapefruit zest, half cup
- Salt, half tsp.
- Lime wedge, two
- Tequila, half cup
- Soda, two cups
- Lime juice, half cup
- Ice cubes, as required

Instructions:
1. Combine the salt, sweetener, and grapefruit zest.
2. Use immediately as it is, or wait ten minutes and then sift out the grapefruit zest before using.
3. Run a wedge of lime or grapefruit around the rim of the glass, and then dip upside down into the salt mixture to coat.
4. Fill the glasses with ice cubes.
5. Pour in the soda, tequila, and lime juice.
6. Stir and serve immediately.

4.12 Keto Tortilla Chips

Cooking Time: 15 minutes

Serving: 4

Ingredients:

- Shredded mozzarella cheese, two cups
- Garlic powder, one tsp.
- Almond flour, one
- Chili powder, one tsp.
- Salt and pepper, as required

Instructions:

1. Line two large baking sheets with parchment paper.
2. In a microwave safe bowl, melt mozzarella, about a minute.
3. Add almond flour, salt, garlic powder, chili powder, and a few cracks black pepper.
4. Using your hands, knead dough a few times until a smooth ball form.
5. Place dough between two sheets of parchment paper and roll out into a rectangle shape.
6. Using a knife or pizza cutter, cut dough into triangles.
7. Spread chips out on prepared baking sheets and bake until edges are golden and starting to crisp.
8. Your dish is ready to be served.

4.13 Keto Queso Dip

Cooking Time: 15 minutes

Serving: 6-8

Ingredients:

- Shredded cheese mix, two cups
- Cream cheese, half cup
- Onions, one
- Jalapeno, one
- Cumin, one tsp.
- Heavy cream, two tbsp.
- Salt and pepper, as required

Instructions:

1. Melt the butter in a skillet over medium heat.
2. Stir in the onion, jalapeno, and cumin and cook for five minutes, or until vegetables are softened.
3. Add the cream cheese, heavy cream, and water to the pan and cook, stirring constantly, over medium heat until the cream cheese melts.

4. Reduce heat to low and add the shredded cheese a handful at a time, whisking constantly, until all of the cheese has been added and the sauce is smooth and creamy.
5. Your dish is ready to be served.

4.14 Keto Guacamole

Cooking Time: 15 minutes
Serving: 4-6
Ingredients:
- Avocados, four
- Garlic, one
- Jalapeno, one
- Sour cream, half cup
- Onion, one
- Lime juice, one tbsp.
- Cilantro, as required
- Tomatoes, one
- Cumin, one tsp.
- Salt and pepper, as required

Instructions:
1. Slice the avocados in half and carefully remove the seed.
2. Scoop the flesh out into a mixing bowl using a spoon.
3. Mash the avocado with a fork to the consistency you prefer.
4. Stir in the sour cream.
5. Dice the tomato and onion.
6. Mince the garlic, jalapeno, and cilantro. Add to the bowl of avocado.
7. Cut the lime in half and squeeze one half of the lime into the bowl.
8. Add the cumin and salt and stir to combine.
9. Taste the guacamole and add more jalapeno, lime juice, and salt.
10. Your dish is ready to be served.

4.15 Keto Soup

Cooking Time: 35 minutes
Serving: 4

Ingredients:

- Chicken broth, three cups
- Water, two cups
- Minced garlic, one tbsp.
- Butter, four tbsp.
- Heavy cream, two cups
- Chopped bacon, half cup
- Chopped kale, two cups
- Onion, half
- Ground sausage, half pound
- Salt and pepper to taste

Instructions:

1. Mix all the ingredients together in a large pot.
2. Cook for thirty-five minutes and then serve hot.

Chapter 5: Keto Mexican Vegetarian Recipes

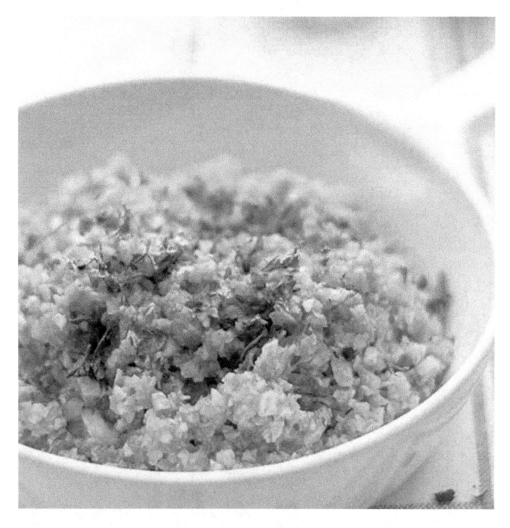

Mexican cuisine is composed of amazing and healthy vegetarian recipes. Following are some recipes that you can easily follow at home:

5.1 Keto Mexican Cauliflower Rice

Cooking Time: 10 minutes

Serving: 4

Ingredients:

- Ground cauliflower, one large
- Mix spice, one tbsp.
- Salt and pepper, to taste
- Vegetable oil, two tbsp.
- Cilantro, as required

Instructions:

1. Add the vegetable oil in a pan
2. Add the shredded cauliflower into it.

3. Add mix spice into the mixture and cook for two minutes.
4. Next, add salt and pepper and cook it for five minutes.
5. Garnish it with cilantro leaves.
6. Your dish is ready to be served.

5.2 Keto Vegetable Soup

Cooking Time: 15 minutes
Serving: 2

Ingredients:

- Salt and pepper, to taste
- Taco seasoning, one tbsp.
- Onion, one
- Minced garlic, three
- Mixed vegetables, two cups
- Tomatoes, one
- Vegetable oil, two tbsp.
- Cilantro, as required
- Vegetable stock, two cups

Instructions:

1. Add the vegetable oil in a large pan and add the onions.
2. Cook the onions and add garlic into it.
3. Next add tomatoes and then the spices.
4. Add the mix vegetables.
5. Add the vegetable stock into the mixture.
6. Let it simmer for ten minutes and then add cilantro on top.
7. Your dish is ready to be served.

5.3 Keto Vegetable Casserole

Cooking Time: 35 minutes
Serving: 4

Ingredients:

- Mixed vegetables, two cups
- Salt and pepper, to taste
- Sour cream, as required
- Onion, one
- Minced garlic, three
- Mixed cheese, one cup
- Avocado, one
- Jalapeno, one
- Taco seasoning, one tbsp.
- Tortillas, nine
- Tomatoes, one

- Mix vegetables, half cup
- Vegetable oil, two tbsp.
- Cilantro, as required

Instructions:
1. Add the vegetable oil and cook the onions in a pan.
2. Then add the garlic and mix vegetables.
3. Cook well and add tomatoes, taco seasoning, salt, and pepper into the mixture.
4. Add the mix vegetables and cook for two minutes.
5. Transfer the mixture into a baking dish and top with cheese blend.
6. Bake it for five minutes.
7. Add the cilantro on top and serve it with tortillas and desired toppings.

5.4 Keto Stuffed Avocados

Cooking Time: 15 minutes

Serving: 6

Ingredients:
- Chopped chives, two tbsp.
- Mix vegetables stuffing, one and a half cup
- Salt and pepper
- Avocado, three
- Vegetable oil, two tbsp.

Instructions:
1. Cut the avocados in half.
2. Remove the seed and your vegetable stuffing in the seed hole.
3. Add the chopped chives on the avocados.
4. Add salt and pepper and bake for ten minutes.
5. Your dish is ready to be served.

5.5 Keto Vegetarian Skillet

Cooking Time: 15 minutes

Serving: 4

Ingredients:
- Mix vegetables, one cup
- Diced bell pepper, half
- Salt and pepper, to taste
- Green chilies, half cup
- Taco seasoning, three tbsp.
- Diced onion, one
- Cauliflower rice, one cup
- Sour cream, as required
- Jalapeno, one
- Tortillas, six

- Avocado one
- Avocado oil, two tbsp.
- Cilantro, as required

Instructions:
1. Heat the avocado oil in a skillet.
2. Add in the mix vegetables and cook.
3. Add in the onion, bell pepper, and taco seasoning and cook for a few minutes or until the onion and pepper start to soften.
4. Stir in the green chilies and tomatoes along with the cauliflower rice.
5. Top with all the toppings.
6. Your dish is ready to be served.

5.6 Keto Vegetarian Enchiladas

Cooking Time: 18 minutes

Serving: 6

Ingredients:
- Mix vegetables, two cups
- Salt and pepper, to taste
- Enchilada sauce, as required
- Onion, one
- Minced garlic, three
- Mixed cheese, one cup
- Avocado, one
- Jalapeno, one
- Tortillas, six
- Tomatoes, one
- Vegetable oil, two tbsp.
- Cilantro, as required

Instructions:
1. Add chopped onions in a pan with the vegetable oil.
2. Once the onions are soft, add the garlic into it.
3. Then, add the mix vegetables into it.
4. Cook for a few minutes and then add tomatoes and let it simmer for five minutes.
5. Add salt and pepper, mix and set aside.
6. Take the tortilla sheets and add the prawn mixture in the center and roll it.
7. Place the rolled tortillas in a baking dish and pour the enchilada sauce over it.
8. Next add the shredded cheese on top.
9. Bake for five minutes until the cheese is melted.
10. Add the cilantro on top and your dish is ready to be served.

5.7 Keto Zucchini Enchiladas

Cooking Time: 35 minutes

Serving: 4

Ingredients:

- Chicken broth, three cups
- Water, two cups
- Minced garlic, one tbsp.
- Butter, four tbsp.
- Heavy cream, two cups
- Chopped bacon, half cup
- Chopped kale, two cups
- Onion, half
- Ground sausage, half pound
- Salt and pepper to taste

Instructions:

5.8 Keto Tomato Soup

Cooking Time: 15 minutes

Serving: 2

Ingredients:
- Salt and pepper, to taste
- Taco seasoning, one tbsp.
- Onion, one
- Minced garlic, three
- Tomatoes, five
- Vegetable oil, two tbsp.
- Cilantro, as required
- Vegetable stock, two cups

Instructions:
1. Add the vegetable oil in a large pan and add the onions.
2. Cook the onions and add garlic into it.
3. Next add tomatoes and then the spices.
4. Add the vegetable stock into the mixture.
5. Let it simmer for ten minutes and then add cilantro on top.
6. Your dish is ready to be served.

5.9 Keto Vegetarian Skewers
Cooking Time: 10 minutes
Serving: 4
Ingredients:
- Wooden skewers, four
- Mix vegetables, two cups
- Cotija and parmesan cheese, half cup
- Chipotle powder, two tsp.
- Salt, as required
- Chopped cilantro, half cup
- Mayonnaise, half cup
- Red sauce, two tsp.

Instructions:
1. Add the mix vegetables in skewers.
2. You can add any vegetable you want.
3. Combine the mayonnaise and red sauce, and then brush generously onto the cauliflower.
4. Sprinkle on all sides with the chipotle powder and salt.
5. Sprinkle or roll in the crumbled cotija or parmesan cheese.
6. Garnish with chopped cilantro.
7. Add the lime juice on top.
8. Your dish is ready to be served.

5.10 Keto Roasted Broccoli
Cooking Time: 15 minutes

Serving: 2

Ingredients:

- Broccoli florets, two cups
- Olive oil, one tbsp.
- Mexican seasoning, one tbsp.
- Salt and pepper to taste

Instructions:

1. Mix all the ingredients together.
2. Keep it in the oven for ten minutes.
3. You can serve it with anything you want.
4. Your dish is ready to be served.

5.11 Keto Vegetarian Cheesy Chili Rellenos

Cooking Time: 15 minutes

Serving: 4

Ingredients:

- Shredded cheese mix, two cups
- Mix vegetable stuffing, one cup
- Raw eggs, two
- Onion powder, half tsp.
- Poblano peppers, eight
- Olive oil, two tbsp.
- Salt and pepper, as required

Instructions:

1. Roast the poblano peppers for five minutes and then stuff it with cheese mix and vegetable stuffing.
2. Beat the eggs until they get fluffy.
3. Next add the spices into the egg mixture.
4. Coat the peppers in the egg mixture.
5. Fry them in olive oil.
6. Your dish is ready to be served with your preferred dip.

5.12 Keto Taco Salad

Cooking Time: 10 minutes

Serving: 4

Ingredients:

- Avocado, one
- Roman lettuce, four cups
- Taco seasoning, three tbsp.
- Parmesan cheese, one cup
- Sour cream, half cup
- Tomato salsa, one cup

- Salt and pepper to taste

Instructions:
1. Mix all the ingredients together.
2. Your dish is ready to be served.

5.13 Keto Zucchini Lasagna

Cooking Time: 15 minutes

Serving: 4

Ingredients:
- Pico de Galo, one cup
- Mix vegetable, one cup
- Mixed vegetables, one cup
- Salt and pepper to taste
- Olive oil, two tbsp.
- Mix cheese, one cup
- Refried beans, one cup
- Cilantro, as required
- Tortilla sheets, eight

Instructions:
1. Add the mix vegetables in a pan and cook for few minutes.
2. Add all the spices and refried beans.
3. Add salt and pepper.
4. Once cooked add the mixture into the tortillas.
5. Add Pico de Galo on top.
6. Roll and place it in a baking tray.
7. Add cheese on top and bake.

5.14 Keto Vegetarian Pizza

Cooking Time: 15 minutes

Serving: 2

Ingredients:
- Shredded cheese mix, two cups
- Cilantro, as required
- Mixed vegetables, one cup
- Jalapenos, two
- Olive oil, two tbsp.
- Salt and pepper, as required

Instructions:
1. Add the cheese on a pan and let it melt.
2. Add the mixed vegetables on top.
3. Add jalapeno peppers on top.
4. Add cilantro and olive oil.

5. Your pizza is ready to be served.

5.15 Keto Vegetarian Burrito

Cooking Time: 15 minutes

Serving: 4

Ingredients:

- Refried beans, one cup
- Mixed vegetables, two cups
- Salt and pepper, to taste
- Hot sauce, as required
- Minced garlic, three
- Mixed cheese, one cup
- Avocado, one
- Jalapeno, one
- Tortillas, four
- Tomatoes, one

Instructions:

1. In the center of each tortilla, spread the refried beans; add mixed vegetables, the taco seasoning, some cheese, and tomato pieces, jalapeno, and avocado.
2. Fold in the two sides and roll up tightly.
3. Lightly fry the burrito.
4. Serve with hot sauce.

5.16 Vegan Keto Walnut Chili

Cooking Time: 30 minutes

Serving: 4

Ingredients:

- Chopped chilies, three
- Chili powder, one tsp.
- Mixed vegetables, two cups
- Onion, one
- Minced garlic, three
- Paprika, one tsp.
- Coriander powder, one tsp.
- Cumin powder, one tsp.
- Tomato paste, half cup
- Vegetable oil, two tbsp.
- Tomatoes, one
- Cilantro, as required
- Walnuts, one cup

Instructions:

1. Place a large saucepan over high heat.

2. Add the oil, onions, garlic and chopped chilis into the pan.
3. Add the chili powder and salt into the pan.
4. Add the vegetables.
5. Add the tomato paste, paprika, cumin and coriander and stir well.
6. Cook for five minutes before adding the canned diced tomatoes.
7. Reduce the heat to a low simmer and continue to cook for twenty to thirty minutes.
8. Taste your chili.
9. Add the walnuts in the end.
10. Add additional salt and pepper if desired.
11. Add cilantro on top.
12. Your dish is ready to be served.

5.17 Keto Cauliflower Tostadas

Cooking Time: 25 minutes
Serving: 6

Ingredients:

- Cauliflower, two cups
- Sweet potato, one cups
- Eggs, two
- Cumin, one tsp.
- Black beans, one cup
- Cilantro, as required
- Coconut oil, two tbsp.
- Avocados, one
- Lime wedges, as required
- Salt and pepper to taste

Instructions:

1. Pulse cauliflower in a food processor until it is completely broken down into couscous-sized granules.
2. Transfer to a bowl and microwave for four minutes, stirring halfway through. Allow to cool, then wrap in a towel or cheesecloth and squeeze to drain out as much liquid as possible.
3. Return cauliflower mixture to a bowl and add eggs, cumin, salt and pepper.
4. Heat a cast iron skillet over medium heat and add coconut oil.
5. Cook cauliflower tostadas until browned on both sides, about two minutes per side.
6. Assemble by spreading a layer of mashed sweet potato over each tostada, followed by avocado and black beans.
7. Season with salt and pepper and garnish with cilantro leaves, hot sauce and a squeeze of lime.

5.18 Keto Vegan Quesadillas
Cooking Time: 10 minutes
Serving: 4

Ingredients:
- Mixed vegetables, two cups
- Butter, two tbsp.
- Salt and pepper to taste
- Mexican spices two tbsp.
- Cheese, one cup
- Tortillas, eight

Instructions:
1. Add the butter in a pan and then add spinach.
2. Add rest of the spices and cook properly.
3. In another pan add the tortillas and add the spinach mixture on top.
4. Then, add the cheese on it.
5. Place another tortilla on top.
6. Cook on both sides.
7. Your dish is ready to be served with your preferred dip.

5.19 Keto Vegan Black Beans and Rice

Cooking Time: three hours

Serving: 4

Ingredients:
- Mexican oregano, one tbsp.
- Soy beans, one cup
- Cauliflower rice, two cups
- Mixed spice, two tsp.
- Vegetable stock, two cups
- Salt and pepper to taste

Instructions:
1. Add everything except the Mexican oregano to your slow cooker and mix around as best as possible.
2. Let it cook on high for about three hours until the rice is tender.
3. Stir in oregano.
4. Garnish as desired and serve immediately.

5.20 Keto Mexican Vegetarian Balls

Cooking Time: 35 minutes

Serving: 4

Ingredients:
- Mixed vegetables, two cups
- Tomato sauce, half cup
- Mexican spice, two tbsp.
- Eggs, one
- Onion, one

- Tomato, one
- Salt and pepper to taste
- Vegetable oil, as required

Instructions:

1. Mix all the things together and make balls.
2. Fry the balls.
3. Your dish is ready to be served with your preferred dip.

Conclusion

Mexican cooking is incredibly vast and amazing. It started from Mexico yet got popular enough to spread worldwide and it was by and by adored and eaten everywhere on the planet. The individuals of the United Stated of America love Mexican food and they devour it consistently.

The purpose for the high ubiquity of the Mexican food is because of the ongoing trend and design of the street food. In this book, we have given 77 distinct recipes of Keto Mexican cuisine that include assorted dishes that you could not imagine anything better than to devour.

The given recipes incorporate solid breakfast, lunch, supper, bites, and vegetarian plans. An individual who does not normally cook, for the most part can undoubtedly make every one of these plans with the definite fixing rundown and simple to adhere directions that are referenced with every recipe in the book. After reading this book, you will be able to better adopt Keto diet by making delicious Keto Mexican recipes at home and become a Mexican chef in no time.

CPSIA information can be obtained
at www.ICGtesting.com
Printed in the USA
LVHW101258010321
679377LV00050B/201

9 781316 209653